MEDICINAL HERBS

TABLE OF CONTENT

INTRODUCTION

Thank you for choosing this book *"Medicinal herbs"*, *A beginner's Guide to Growing and Using Herbs for Both Medicinal and Culinary Purposes.*

Medicinal herbs have been used since the beginning of human history as a source of food to increase strength, cure different types of disorders and improve overall health. Herb is one of the most prehistoric of the healing arts. It's the medicine of the people and always will be. Not even all the regulatory measures put in place by the FDA can prevent people from benefiting from these gifts of nature. Herbal plants have been in existence long before human. They have learnt to adapt to their surroundings and have provided simple language to communicate those lessons with other plants, animals and other natural creature.

The word "herb" was derived from an old French word "herbe" and the Latin word "herba". Today, a herb is referred to as any part of the medicinal plant such as root, stigma, leaf, flower, bark, stem, seed and fruit as well as non-woody plants. These medicinal plants are not only used as food, medicine, perfume, and flavonoid, but are also used in some specific spiritual activities.

This book is written to provide you with adequate information on how to grow, harvest, prepare and use these amazing plants to improve your health and overall well-being.

Thanks again for choosing this book. I hope you find all the information helpful.

CHAPTER 1

What is Medicinal Herb?

Herbal medicines are plant-based medications made from different combinations of plant parts such as roots, seeds, fruits, flowers, or leaves. Every single part could have varied medicinal uses and the different kinds of chemical components require different extraction techniques. Both dried and fresh plant matter is used, depending on the herb.

Medicinal herb is the oldest and still the most universally used method of medication in the present world. Its medicine is made wholly from plants. It is being used by every culture and is commonly found in every society.

You might often notice medicinal plants being referred to as natural remedies, alternative medicine, phytomedicine or botanical medicine. Medicinal herb is the employ of the energetic and chemical compounds in a plant's roots, stems, berries, flowers, and leaves to influence the body and enhance healing.

Treatment with herbal plants is regarded as harmless as there are little or no side effects. The significant advantage is that these remedies are in line with nature. The golden truth is that the use of herbal remedies is independent of any sexes and age groups.

The prehistoric researchers are of the opinion that herbal medicines are the   only solutions to cure numerous health-related diseases and conditions. A thorough study was conducted to arrive at precise conclusions about the effectiveness of several herbs with medicinal value. The majority of the medicines thus formulated are free of reactions or side effects. This is the rationale behind the growth in popularity of herbal treatment all over the world. These herbal plants with medicinal value provide rational means for treating several internal ailments that are otherwise considered not easy to be cured.

CHAPTER 2

Forms of Medicinal Herb

Medicinal herb could be provided in various ways. The medicine form adopted would be determined by the part of the plants to be accessed, individual, age, and their conditions of health. Medicinal herb can be used in the following forms:

- Capsules

- Compress

- Herbal Tea

- Essential Oils

- Tincture

- Syrups

- Elixirs

- Glycerites

- Suppositories

- Poultice

- Oils

- Salves

SAFETY PRECAUTIONS

Medicinal herb is all-natural but might not always be entirely safe. Many herbs are wonderfully tolerated and categorized as safe to be consumed in the Botanical Safety Handbook of the American Herbal Product Association (AHPA). Nevertheless, there are varieties of herbs used by herbalist that necessitate precise dosage and preparation consideration for every single individual. Drug and herb interaction might also be considered when using medicinal herb along with pharmaceutical medicines. For this reasons, it's pertinent to work with a certified and qualified herbalist or a doctor that has vast knowledge in the use of medicinal herbs

CHAPTER 3

Medicinal Herb in History

Herbs have been in use since primeval periods. Ancient Greeks and Romans crowned their emperors with laurel and dill. The Romans also make use of dill to cleanse the air. Hippocrates, the famous Greek physician, itemized about four hundred herbs commonly in use in the 5th century. About 65 A.D., a Greek physician (called Pedanius Dioscorides) serving with the Roman warriors, wrote "De Materia Medica" where he described the medicinal values of several herbs. Up till today, it's regarded as one the most prominent herbal books.

In the Middle Ages, people used herbs to preserve meat and also to cover the decaying taste of meals that could not be refrigerated. They also used herbs to neutralize the odors of the people who don't bathe regularly. These periods were unfavorable to the evolution of herbs in medicine. The Catholic Church started killing herbalists as they were associated with both paganism and witchcraft. Most of the early settlers cultivated herbs for their medicinal properties and for seasoning their food. Indian American often used of herbs for dyeing and tanning leather.

There are 3 major medicinal herbs traditions that derived from the use of herbs in prehistory age

1. Western

Based on Roman and Greek sources, The Romans and Greeks hypothesized that four humors pervaded the body and that these liquids and their relations affected the health. Every single fluid – phlegm, blood, yellow bile, and black bile – was linked with one of the similar 4 nature's elements respectively – water, fire, earth, and air. Greco-Roman civilization, this medical philosophy was passed on to the European countries where it passed on through the Middle Ages. And it began gaining approval in the renaissance period.

Back in the days of the Roman Empire, the only available medications were predominantly herbs and other natural therapies. Though patients could consult physicians, commonly health care began with treatment devised by the household's heads. They would treat members of the family and servants with concoctions such as wine or vinegar for wounds disinfection. Puppy juice, mixed with the yolk of an egg and eggshell ash, was dysentery "remedy". Roman physicians and surgeons used henbane seeds (scopolamine) and extracts of opium (morphine) as a painkiller.

Evidently, there have been changes on the concept of illnesses over the times. While Galen, the Greek physician used buckthorn (Rhamnus fragula) to protect patients against demons and witches in the second century, nowadays Buckthorn is most commonly used as a laxative. Consequently, the application might have changed; numerous herbal medicines are still in use. For instance, anise was used by Hippocrates to treat coughs, even up till the present time the treatment still in existence.

2. Ayurvedic

Ayurveda or Ayurvedic medicine (from India), is a holistic approach to therapeutic that was initiated in India about 1500 B.C. It emphasizes that an individual's well-being is the consequence of a natural balance and that the occurrence of illness is a result of imbalance. Natural remedies and herbs are to reinstate balance.

3. Traditional Chinese

Traditional Chinese Medicine (TCM), dating back about two thousand to three thousand years, is based on a belief that your well-being is the consequence of constant battling between opposing forces (yang and yin). If these forces are imbalance, you fall sick. When they are in balance, you will be in good health condition. Therapies are aimed to stimulate the body's curing machinery and include, among other things, herbal medicines and moxibustion (burning herbs near skin). The United State National Library of Medicine embraces about two thousand volumes of Chinese medical classics.

While most of our present herbal medicines derived from the Greek, Roman, Chinese, and Ayurvedic sources all ancient civilizations, comprising the

Egyptian, Aztecs, and Mayans adopted herbs in treating illnesses. For instance, an Egyptian housewife that had a sore throat would treat it by gargling with a combination of vinegar and garlic. It would give her an additional benefit of minty fresh breath.

CHAPTER 4

Growing Medicinal Plants

Discover the numerous rewards of growing medicinal herbs. Grow medicinal herbs and plants in your home and start enjoying the rewards of medicinal herbs. Though several homesteaders embrace medicinal herbs, not everybody understands how great these herbal remedies work, and how they can be well grown on their own land.

The main impediment is that many people still attach superstition to medicinal herb, thinking it is all mythology without proven worth. However, if the statement is true, it will be a surprise to the large pharmaceutical companies that are scrambling to separate and test the active elements of many traditional medicinal herbs and plants. Numerous powerful pharmaceuticals, for instance, have been derived from wild yam. Meadowsweet and willow have salicylic acidic with analgesic properties such as aspirin – with lesser side effects though. Controlled researches of valerian have upheld its traditional use as a sedative to induce sleep and relief spasms.

The other impediment to the domestic use of herbal medicine is just the opposite – the belief that herbal tradition is so secretive that the inexperienced homesteaders may not likely to master it without years of learning. In this case, I suggest you look at various common herbal medicines in the below list. These herb lists are cited from the California School of Herbal Studies.

Most of these herbs and plant are renowned, and might already be growing in your garden or backyard comfrey, chamomile, calendula, and black cherry – who thought these unobtrusive and ubiquitous members of our societies would make" top thirty" list of herbal medicines.

A number of these are weeds. We have been made to think of yellow dock, stinging nettle, plantain and dandelion as "the antagonist" in our yards and gardens. Maybe it is time to change our perception toward weeds. I mean we should start perceiving plants and herbs as part of our local ecosystem by exploring its contribution and role, rather than finding means of eradicating them. Any plant or herb that provides improvements to our health should be embraced and honored, instead of degraded as a weed.

CHAPTER 5

Benefits of Growing Medicinal Plants

Growing medicinal plants provide numerous benefits to humans, plants and the environments, the following are some the benefits of growing medicinal plants in your garden.

- **Herbal medicinal as foods**

As earlier mentioned, most of the plants we have come to depend on for food also has medicinal values. The food part in some cases differing from the therapeutic part – for instance, it's often the blackberry root bark that is being used for medicinal purposes. But in most cases, it's the edible part of the plants that we consume as food, balancing and toning the body while adding spices to our meals, like peppermint, ginger, fennel, and cayenne (a common digestive and circulatory system tonic). We ought to integrate such herbs more regularly into our diets and discover their use in a more formal way when the need arises. For example, we could make an infusion of fennel to stimulate appetite or digestion, or to treat colic.

- **Herbs could be used to prepare other foods with medicinal effects.**

During the ancient periods, a variety of herbal plants – berries, elderflowers, St. John's wort, licorice, wintergreen, ginger, and yarrow were used to flavor and preserve ales and beers. Vegetable oils and vinegar can be infused with herbs such as cayenne, garlic, and rosemary, and served on salad and other meals to improve our health. Mead, a fermented drink made from honey, has its medicinal values, but could also be prepared with herbs like heather to boost its medicinal richness.

- **Herbs to Boost Insect Diversity**

Experienced homesteaders are aware that the solution to managing insects isn't a process for killing them, but allowing even more insect diversity, mainly by growing plants flower all through the growing seasons. Numerous common herbal medicines – such as Echinacea, yarrow, calendula, fennel, peppermint, and chamomile – are flowering plants, and also have the value of providing food and shelter to the beneficiaries. Growing of flowering plants and herbs are more effective at boosting our insect allies when integrated with the crops to be protected, instead of planting them separately.

- **Herbs as fertility plants**

Clever homesteaders are also aware that we can grow more of our soil fertility. Fortunately enough, a number of the best fertility plants also possess medicinal properties. Comfrey – used for healing broken bones and wounds - and nettle are rich in protein and could be used to "spark" a compost heap or as nutritive mulches. Yellow dock and dandelion are deep-rooted active collectors that mine mineral deposits from the sub-soil and offering them to more shallow-rooted crops

- **Herbs as fodder crops**

A large number of medicinal herbs and plants perform dual functions of providing dried fodder or fresh green for our livestock. I discovered that yellow duck and dandelion remain green deeper into winter's cold than other forage plans – I dig them up and feed to my flocks. Oats could be used to feed livestock and also make a wonderful nerve tonic. Either self-harvested or cut and fed green. My geese love comfrey

- **Other landscape or ecological uses**

Willow and hawthorn may be cultivated as a living fence, as a windbreak or for shade. As much as they provide essential environmental benefits – Wildlife and bird shelter and moderation of the wind effects, heat and loss of soil humidity to evaporation – in addition to their therapeutic values.

CHAPER 6

Useful Tips on Cultivation

You can grow your own medicinal herbs just about anywhere. There are traditional medicinal herbs and plants on the homestead to suit any micro-ecology. For instance, the drier, more open segment of the homestead could be planted with lemon balm, clary, sage, thyme, rue, lavender, hyssop, rosemary, milk thistle, chaste berry. Moister areas could accommodate angelica, scullcap, goldenrod, cardinal flower, selfheal, peppermint, and mullein.

I cultivated a woodland garden of culinary and medicinal herbs in a fold of small woodlot, which is more probable of staying damp than any other setting in my area. Shade-loving herbs such as goldenseal – a key medicinal plant of many Native American tribes, an important antimicrobial for acute infections-, blue cohosh, black cohosh, wild yam, spikenard, wild ginger, Solomon's seal, downy rattlesnake, and bloodroot all grow well there.

You might have heard that herbs love to grow in poor soil. The fact is that most herbs don't have the high nitrogen necessities of heavy feeders such as squash and corn, all plants choose to grow in soil that it nurtured and loved. As it's applicable in the rest of the garden, make every effort to improve the organic matter in your soil. Growing cover crops, using mulches, adding composts, and your medicinal plantings would thrive well.

Some medicinal plants also could be found in the wild, but unluckily a lot are endangered by overharvesting. Experienced herbalists shun wildcrafting of threatened herbal types – and in reality, it helps in preserving these priceless parts of our environmental heritage by propagating and growing herbs such as bloodroot, American ginseng, black cohosh, pipsissewa, and goldenseal.

CHAPTER 7

How to Make Herbal Medications

Make your kitchen your pharmacy. Get the necessary equipment such as measuring utensils, funnel, filters, electric coffee grinder, pans, and bowls. Let them be available in your kitchen. To make more sophisticated extractions, you can include items like distilling and presses equipment.

With a reliable beginner's guide to home medicine, you would be surprised that you could duplicate by yourself all the forms that you've encountered drugs before. Tinctures (based on wine, vinegar, glycerin, and even alcohol), infusions (medicinal herbs could be as simple as a cup of coffee) and lotions, salves, syrups, tablets, and decoctions. Also, some that may be new to you such as fomentations, poultices, and herbal water baths.

Traditional herbalist almost regularly makes use of the entire plant or their extracts as medication. Modern pharmaceutical prefers to single out an element of a plant as the "active ingredient," and administering the singled-out component from other composites. Perhaps, this could be the single rational behind the increased occurrence of accidental side effects of modern medications, and their vastly higher cost. The complementary composites of the entire plant will not only help alleviate side-effects and balance its action, but also evidently help "nourish" our vital intestinal flora, and consequently act as a useful pro-biotic in the digestive tract.

SAFETY TIPS ON MAKING HERBAL MEDICINE

The fact that medicinal herbs are natural doesn't imply they could be taken without considering the possible dangers. A number of our potential herb buddies are somewhat powerful indeed and could be hazardous if misused. The following important safety rules will help for the safe use of medicinal plants and herbs.

1. **Know the plant**

Appropriate identification of plant is essential – there is no room for guessing games or carelessness. Fennel is a common herbal medicine, and other allied species like cilantro, dill, lovage, celery, and parsley also have a long history of medicinal use. However, one of the two related plant species may be poisonous for example; poison hemlock and water hemlock, any mistake with these similar plants could be deadly. This may sound frightening, but we just need to be attentive and careful so as not to select wrong plants or herbs.

2. Know what part of the plant to be used

It is possible that one part of a medicinal plant or herb is safe to be used, while others are not consumable. For instance, berries and elderberry flowers are safe to use for the beginners (to make medications for fever and flu), but the bark may have poisonous properties.

3. Understand the application

Some plants could be safe to use externally but could be very toxic if consumed internally. A perfect example is digitalis (foxglove), which could be deadly if consumed but could be used in making fomentation to help wound healing.

4. Understand the dosage

We should never assume the same dosage for every individual and in every circumstance. Indeed, James Green notices that smaller dosages of German chamomile can offer positive results for the nervous system, in which larger dosages can't do. In most cases, the probability of toxicity or side effects rises with increasing dose. Keep in mind the dose also affect the body weight. Thus, we must take proper care when giving medicinal herbs to children.

5. Know the possible side effects

Although undesirable side effects are much less common in medicinal herbs than in pharmaceuticals, it's advisable that you read and understand herbal literature to lessen probable side effects. For instance, herbs high in tannins like yellow dock (a laxative and liver stimulant) could be problematic for people that have a history of kidney stone.

6. Take cognizance of individual sensitivities

A person may have an allergic reaction to a particular herbal medicine safely taken by others. Thus when starting the use of any herbal medicine, begin with a lesser dosage and work up to a standard dosage.

7. **Be conscious of usage restrictions**

Some safe to use medicinal plants by the general individual might not be suitable for the aged or children. Most significantly, pregnant women should always be given special consideration. When we talk of any medicinal plant, an experienced herbalist would put into an account, the issue of safe use during pregnancy and would not stumble on the part of cautiousness. Some herbs like yarrow, mugwort, goldenseal, comfrey, and black cohosh should not be taken by pregnant women at all. Others plants like ginger and cayenne may be taken, but very carefully.

8. Know your own expertise limits

Numerous herbal medicines are safe and comfortable for a beginner to consume. It is ideal to begin with, herbs commonly taken in tea or as food. Other may require far greater knowledge, skill, and experience. For example, elderberry bark stated above, is indeed an excellent medicinal herb, even for internal uses. But it's powerful and ought to be prescribed by the experienced and knowledgeable herbalist. The rest of us should make do with the more natural to use herbs and consult a reliable expertise if there is need for advancement.

You might found as you honor and get to understand medicinal plants, cultivated and wild, that your affiliation with these herbs grows ever more personal, more intimate. Medicinal herb is not only about making use of plants and herbs to make compounds we equate one-for-one with illness symptom. While chemical plants produce could truly be healing, our rising relationships with plants are even more so.

CHAPTER 8

5 Medicinal Herbs for a Healthy Brain

Most herbs and spices have medicinal benefits, and some of them are found to enhance brain health. Aim to get more of these in particular.

1. Turmeric

The yellow mustard powder is a powerful anti-inflammatory and an antioxidant. The risk of developing Alzheimer's is 25 percent in India where turmeric is being consumed daily in curries, lower than the risk in the United State. Integrating these with other daily routines that prevent Alzheimer's into your life might further increase your likelihoods of preventing the disease. Rats that consumed the central element in turmeric in the lab studies, got fewer amyloid plaques, related to Alzheimer's, than mice that were not. Scientific studies have also established a direct link between the herb and brain health. You can add turmeric to egg salad, to any curry dish or add about a teaspoonful in lentils, casseroles or pea soup. Try turmeric for a Creole skillet dinner, and look for more lip-smacking recipes that could boost brain power.

2. Wasabi

A mustard family member, this is the green condiment prepared with sushi. This is an exceptional source of a composite that aids the growth of nerve cells extensions known as axons and dendrites that enhance cells communication with one another. You can see wasabi as a powder or in a tube at specialty stores. Add a little amount to peanut-based sauces or ginger-teriyaki to serve fish with wasabi mayo, crab cakes, coleslaw, salad green, and deviled eggs.

3. Garlic

Garlic can slightly lessen cholesterol without drugs and helps thin blood to prevent blood clots. It possesses compounds that protect neurons from diseases and injury by enhancing the chemicals that cells need to withstand stress. Put tablespoon of pulverized garlic to salad dressing or any marinade. Add stir-fried garlic to vegetable dishes, pasta, tofu, pork, beef, or chicken. Begin with this recipe for Buttery Garlic Potatoes.

4. Parsley and Thyme

Thyme and Parsley are both contain a plant compound known as apigenin. The compound was applied to the human stem cells by the Brazilian researchers and the outcomes seem promising. The stem cells formed neurons which established more sophisticated and stronger connections between them. Researchers hope that their findings would trigger new treatment for diseases such as depression and Alzheimer's. Use thyme and parsley to cook. Select from Thyme Butternut Squash.

5. Rosemary

Perceiving the aroma of rosemary alone can boost your brain. A study in the journal Therapeutic Advances in Psychopharmacology established that partakers were more accurate and faster on cognitive tests when snuffling an essential oil of rosemary. A further survey linked camosic acid; the active rosemary ingredient can also safeguard the brain against free radicals to avoid neuron-degeneration and stroke.

CHAPTER 9

20 Herbs You Can Use in Recipes

The following are some common herbs and their culinary uses and the vegetable, dishes, and foods they enhance.

- **Herb**: Basil

Scientific name: (Ocimum basilicum)

Basil is exceptional with cauliflower, green beans, wax beans, corn, herb sandwiches, meatloaf, spaghetti, dips, tuna, salmon, eggs dishes, chicken dishes, salad dressing, pizza, salad, soup, and tomatoes.

- **Herb**: Bay leaves

Scientific name: (Laurus nobilis)

Bay leaves are great with soups, sauce, terrines, pate, garnish, syrups, stocks, casseroles, pickling, steamed fish, stews, and meats.

- **Herb**: Chervil

Scientific name: (Anthriscus cerefolium)

Chervil is good with cottage cheese, herb butter, fish, chicken, soups, vegetables, salads, and eggs

Herb: Chives

Scientific name: (Allium schoenoprasum)

Chives are superb in herb sandwiches, vichyssoise, soups, carrots, salads, cheese soufflés, egg dishes, baked and mashed potatoes barbecues, cold chicken, garnish, sauces, spreads, and dip

- **Herb**: Cilantro

Scientific name: (Coriandrum sativum)

Cilantro goes with beans, dips, soups, chutneys, salsas, stews, guacamole, and salads, used in Asian, Indian, Mexican, Caribbean, and North African cuisines.

- **Herb**: Coriander

Scientific name: (Coriandrum sativum)

Coriander can be used in apple crumble recipes, tea cakes, fruit puddings, fish, veal, pickles, Asian cooking, Greek dishes, Indian dishes, curry, and ginger cookies.

- **Herb**: Dill weed

Scientific name: (Anethum graveolens)

Dill weed is excellent with cabbage, wax beans, green beans, egg and cheese dishes, bread and sandwiches, vinegar and oils, fish dishes, seafood and shellfish, vegetable stews, soups, sauces, dips, herb butter, and salads. Dill seeds are good in bread, cakes, teas, coleslaw, and pickling.

- **Herb**: Fennel

Scientific name: (Foeniculum vulgare)

Fennel is delightful with sauces, salad dressings stuffing /dressings, flavored butter, veal, pork, duck, fish, and salads. Its seed is used in bread.

- **Herb**: Lemongrass

Scientific name: (Cymbopogon citratus)

Lemongrass is used in Asian and Caribbean dishes (Thai and Vietnamese), beef, seafood, fish, tomatoes, chicken, stir fry, sauces, and soups.

- **Herb**: Mint

Scientific name: (Mentha)

Mint can be used in sauces, mint jelly, mint juleps, cold drinks, tea, vegetables such as buttered peas, desserts (mmm ice cream), garnish, mint ice, mashed potatoes, egg dishes, herb sandwiches, soft cheeses, pea soup, lamb sauce, and carrot.

- **Herb**: Oregano

Scientific name: (Origanum vulgare)

Oregano is commonly used in tomatoes sauces, pates and poultry dishes, pizza, Italian dishes, bread, casseroles, soups, (tomatoes, pea), and goes great with salads, vegetables, cabbage, rice, beans, egg dishes, and veal

- **Herb**: Parsley

Scientific name: (Petroselinum crispum)

Parsley is perfect in salads dips, Meat and fish sauces, bread and sandwiches, omelets and other egg dishes soups (tomatoes, fish, vegetables), garnishes, salad dressing, potatoes, tuna loaf, hamburgers, stuffing, and sausage,

- **Herb**: Rosemary

Scientific name: (Rosmarinus officinalis)

Rosemary is palatable in stews, liver pate, dressings, dumplings, bread and scones, vegetables particularly cauliflower, beef and mutton stock, lamb, chicken and poultry sauces.

- **Herb**: Sage

Scientific name: (Salvia officinalis)

Sage is good in meatloaf, meatballs, Brussels sprouts, salads, vegetarian stews, omelets, casseroles, sausage, duck, goose, fish, pizza, Welsh rabbit, pork, sauces, soup (chicken, minestrone), and stuffing/ dressing

- **Herb**: Savory

Scientific name: (Satureja)

Savory is super in hamburger, condiments, stuffing/ dressing, eggs, lentils, soups, dried bean dishes, vegetables, and add spices to gravy.

- **Herb**: Sorrel

Scientific name: (Rumex scutatus)

Sorrel is palatable in goat cheese, white meats, poultry eggs, fish, vegetables, salads, white and cream sauces, and in cold soup.

- **Herb**: Sweet Marjoram

Scientific name: (Origanum majorana)

Sweet marjoram is excellent in fruit salads, stews, cheese and egg dishes, sauces, salads, soups, stuffing/ dressing, and in dishes with peas.

- **Herb**; Tarragon

Scientific name: (Artemisia dracunculus)

Tarragon add spices to cottage cheese, butter, vegetables (cauliflower and green beans in particular), vinegars and oils, salad dressings, sauces, cream and butter, mayonnaise, green salads, egg dishes, seafood, pate, liver, meats, mushrooms, tarragon tartare sauce (tartar sauce), fish sauce and soups, as well as chicken.

- **Herb**: Thyme

Scientific name: (Thymus vulgaris)

Thyme adds spices to cottage cheese, butter, tomatoes, lentil stew, vinegar and oils, beans, broccoli, egg dishes, chicken, stuffing, rabbit, braised, meatballs, pate, liver, soup (vegetables and chicken), beef broth, fish and chicken marinades, salads, cheeses, and chowders.

CHAPTER 10

Over 60 Common Medicinal Plants and Their Uses

The following is the list of some of the more widely known herbs and how you can use them to improve many facets of your health. As I have said earlier, do not to start any course of herbal, treatment or otherwise, without first consulting physician or other healthcare specialists. Ensure you talk over any previously used medications, as herbs could have damaging interactions with other medicines.

- **Herb**: Agrimony

Scientific Name: Agrimonia eupatoria

Family: Rosaceae

Common Names: Common agrimony, stickle-wort or church steeples

Useful Part: Aerial parts

Habitation: Agrimony is indigenous to Europe, but could also be found in the moderate climate in most parts of the Northern hemisphere.

This medicinal herb tea is soothing and good for sore throats. Singers sometimes used it to gargle. Agrimony is used to clear and refresh the throat. It could be used internally for skin sores. The herb can also be prescribed for fevers, asthma and coughs, as well as digestive and bowel problems.

PRECAUTION: Agrimony might make the skin more sensitive to sunlight and this might add to the danger of sunburn. Thus it should not be taken by pregnant women or nursing mother, and people planning to undergo surgery within ttwo weeks.

- **Herb**: Alfalfa

Scientific Name: Medicago sativa

Family: Fabaceae

Common Names: Lucerne, Chilean clover, and Buffalo grass

Useful Part: Sprouts, stems, and leaves.

Habitation: Alfalfa is indigenous to Southeastern Europe and Southwestern Asia. Also grows in North African and American.

This medicinal plant is rich in protein, minerals, and vitamins. Alfalfa roots go down deep as far as thirty feet to draw valuable nutrients from the soil. It is generally used for digestive problems, reducing high cholesterol, as a diuretic, and for arthritis. Alfalfa also has chlorophyll which is useful for reducing body odor and bad breath. The herb is also rich in beta-carotene and an immune system booster.

PRECAUTION: Alfalfa seeds are not safe for consumption since they contain high levels of the amino acid canavanine. Also, it includes stachydrine and homostachydrine which are not good for pregnant women and nursing mother.

- **Herb**: Aloe

Scientific Name: Aloe Vera

Family: Asphodelaceae

Common Names: Aloe, Barbados, cape

Useful Part: Leaves

Habitation: Aloe is indigenous to the Mediterranean. It also grows in the Caribbean and Latin America.

The gel of this medicinal plant is suitable for moisturizing the skin and is among the ingredients of many skin care products. Aloe Vera gel could be used internally to treat poison ivy, scrapes, cuts, sunburn, and minor burns. It can also be used to ease acne and treat several other skin diseases.

PRECAUTION; Aloe should not be used internally as a laxative, as it's unsafe and can result in diarrhea, severe cramping and dangerous imbalances of electrolytes.

- **Herb**: American Ginseng

Scientific Name: Panax quinquefolius

Family: Araliaceae

Common Names: Xi yang shen, ginseng

Useful Part: Root

Habitation: American Ginseng grows in Canada and the eastern part of North America.

This medicinal herb has been used to increase strength and stamina, strengthen the immune system, treat ADHD, diabetes, digestive disorder, and as a tonic for overall wellness. American ginseng is known as cooling herb, while the Korean ginseng has a warming impact on the body system. Generally, ginseng is good for the body and protects against any stress.

PRECAUTION: American Ginseng should not be consumed by pregnant women and people with high blood pressure.

- **Herb**: Amla

Scientific Name: Phyllanthus emblica

Family: Phyllanthaceae

Common Names: Indian gooseberry

Useful Part: Fruit

Habitation: Amla is indigenous to India

This medicinal plant is used in the Ayurvedic herbals system of India. It contains antioxidants and minerals, rich in vitamin C and also has several other vitamins. Phyllanthus emblica is often used to control blood sugar, treat urinary tract infection, fevers, and inflammation of the joints.

- **Herb**: Angelica

Scientific Name: Angelica archangelica

Family: Apiaceae

Common Names: Norwegian angelica, masterwort, holy ghost, wild celery, garden angelica,

Useful part: Roots Leaves, seeds, stems

Habitation: Angelica grows in the Eastern U.S., Asia, and Europe

This medicinal plant has been used traditionally for arthritis, respiratory ailments, digestive problems, appetite loss, flatulence, and menopausal troubles. Just like its Chinese counterpart Angelica Sinensis, Angelica is used by women for the reproductive system. It's known for being a uterine tonic and hormonal regulator.

PRECAUTION: Angelica is not safe to be consumed during pregnancy.

- **Herb**: Anise

Scientific Name: Pimpinella anisum

Family: Umbelliferae

Common Names: Anise

Useful Part: Seeds

Habitation: Anise is indigenous to Egypt

This medicinal herb can be used to treat coughs, reduce bad breath, prevent flatulence, and to improve digestion. Anise tea is made from the seed of the plant and has a strong licorice taste.

- **Herb**: Arnica

Scientific Name: Arnica montana

Family: Asteraceae

Common Names: Mountain arnica, mountain daisy, leopard's bane

Useful Part: Flowers

Habitation: Arnica is native to Europe, Siberia, and central Asia, cultivated in North America.

This medicinal plant is used externally as an ointment for bruises, sprains and sore muscles. It has antiseptic, anti-inflammatory and analgesic properties.

PRECAUTION: Arnica is not recommended for long-term use as it might result in skin irritation. It should not be used internally.

- **Herb**: Ashwagandha

Scientific Name: Withania Somnifera

Family: Solanaceae

Common Names: Indian ginseng, ajagandha, winter cherry

Useful Part: Seeds, leaves, roots

Habitation: Ashwagandha is native to Africa and India and widely cultivated across the globe.

This medicinal herb is well-liked in Indian Ayurvedic herbals system. It is commonly used to boost the immune system and relieve stress. Ashwagandha has been used in India for more than three thousand years as a rejuvenator. It seeds are known to contain diuretic effect, while the leaf has sedative, analgesic and anti-inflammatory components. The root's chemical elements have an immune strengthening, analgesic, sedative, anti-inflammatory, and anti-microbial properties. This herb is good for athletes and those that need to improve their strength, stamina, and energy.

PRECAUTION: Ashwagandha may have a mild depressant effect, thus do not take with alcohol and sedative. Its iron content is also high and should not be consumed by pregnant women.

- **Herb**: Astragalus

Scientific Name: Astragalus membranaceus

Family: Fabaceae

Common Names: Milk vetch, yellow leader, Huang Qi

Useful Part: Roots, rhizomes

Habitation: Astragalus is native to China and Mongolia, cultivated in Canada and the U.S.

This medicinal herb is among the most popular herbs in the Chinese traditional system of medicine. It has been in use for more than two thousand years. Astragalus is most often used for regulating high pressure and as a diuretic. It's also commonly used to treat cold, upper respiratory infection, diarrhea, ulcers, excessive sweating and also to boost the immune system as well as to increase energy.

- **Herb**: Bacopa

Scientific Name: Bacopa Monnieri

Family: Scrophulariaceae

Common Names: Water hyssop, Thyme-leafed gratiola, Coastal Waterhyssop, Brahmi

Useful Part: Whole plant.

Habitation: Bacopa is native to India

This medicinal herb has been used in the Indian Ayurvedic system of medication as an effective brain tonic for thousands of years. It's beneficial to short and long-term memory. The bacosides and saponins found in the plant have a positive impact on the brain's neurotransmitters and could help people to think faster. The plant is currently being studied as a potential treatment for Parkinson's, ADHD, and Alzheimer's disease. It can also be used to treat bronchitis, allergies, asthma, anxiety, and depression.

- **Herb**: Bearberry

Scientific Name: Arctostaphylos uva-ursi

Family: Ericaceae

Common Names: Bear's Grape, uva ursi, kinnikinnick, mountain box

Useful Part: Leaves

Habitation: Bearberry grows all through the Northern Hemisphere

This medicinal herb is usually consumed as a tea, and it's commonly used to treat inflammatory of the urinary tract and urinary tract infections. Bearberry possess antiseptic, diuretic and astringent properties

PRECAUTION: High doses of bearberry could be toxic. It should not be taken by pregnant women, children and those with kidney disease.

- **Herb**: Bee Balm

Scientific Name: Monarda didyma

Family: Lamiaceae

Common Names: Scarlet bergamot, mountain mint, Oswego tea

Useful Part: Leaves

Habitation: Bee Balm is indigenous to North America

This medicinal plant is commonly used by Native Americans to cure flatulent, colic, and intestinal problems. Tea made from bee balm is often used to cure fever and induce sweating. This herb is regularly used to treat a sore throat and a common cold. Its leaf is a good source of essential oil that has thymol, which is an antibiotic and also one of the mouthwash ingredients.

- **Herb**: Bilberry

Scientific Name: Vaccinium mytilus

Family: Ericaceae

Common Names: Whortleberry, European blueberry, huckleberry

Useful Part: Leaves, fruits

Habitation: Bilberry grows in the warm areas of the Northern Hemisphere

This medicinal herb has been used for centuries by European herbalist to treat ailments such as diabetes, diarrhea and stomach pains. Bilberry is now commonly used to prevent night blindness. It's also capable of strengthening the capillaries and guards them against free radical injury. This herb has flavonoids known as anthocyanosides, which are a strong antioxidant.

- **Herb**: Black Cherry

Scientific Name: Prunus serotina

Family: Rosaceae

Common Names: Rum cherry bird cherry,

Useful Part: Bark

Habitation: Black Cherry is indigenous to North America

This medicinal herb is used by the Native Americans to treat coughs. Its bark possesses a glycoside known as prunasin - the substance that ease spasms in the smooth muscle of the bronchioles, therefore lessening the reflex of coughs. The black cherry tree's bark made as syrup or tea has been used to heal the ulcer, expel worm, treat burns, sore throat, and pneumonia as well as a remedy for loss of appetite.

- **Herb**: Black Cohosh

Scientific Name: Cimicifuga racemosa

Family: Ranunculaceae

Common Names: Bugbane, bugwort, macrotys, black snakeroot

Useful Part: Rhizome, roots

Habitation: Black Cohosh is indigenous to North America

This medicinal herb has been used by the Native Americans to treat sore throats, rheumatism, and menstrual irregularities. The Cherokee Indians have also used it as a remedy for tuberculosis and fatigue as well as a diuretic. In recent times, black cohosh has been mainly used to minimize the severity of premenopausal and menopausal symptoms, like hot flashes, depression and excessive sweating.

PRECAUTION: Black cohosh and blue cohosh are not the same. Blue cohosh has not been confirmed to be safe for consumption, thus it may be toxic.

- **Herb**: Boneset

Scientific Name: Eupatorium perfoliatum

Family: Compositae

Common Names: Sweat plant, agueweed, feverwort, Indian Sage

Useful Part: Flowers and leaves

Habitation: Boneset is indigenous to North America

This medicinal herb was used by the Native Americans to induce sweating and to treat flu, indigestion, arthritis, and colds. It is also good for curing malaria, typhoid, constipation, cholera, dengue, and loss of appetite. Boneset is still in use today to treat, flu, colds and minor inflammation.

PRECAUTION: Boneset might cause diarrhea, nausea, and vomiting if a large amount is taken. Do not consume fresh boneset as its toxic Dry it before consumption. It is not safe to be taken by breastfeeding mother, pregnant woman, and people who are allergic to ragweed.

- **Herb**: Borage

Scientific Name: Borago officinalis

Family: Boraginaceae

Common Names: Talewort, bee Plant, Burrage, star flower, beebread

Useful Part: Flowers, seed oil

Habitation: Borage is indigenous to Southern Europe

This medicinal plant is commonly used as a diuretic, to treat inflammation of mucous membranes, lung infection, and fever. Borage is also effective as a sedative and mild anti-depressant. The oil from its seeds are loaded with gamma-linolenic acid (GLA).which is a fatty acid that fights inflammation and boosts body immunity.

- **Herb**: Boswellia

Scientific Name: Boswellia serrata

Family: Burseraceae

Common Names: Salai guggul, Indian olibanum dhup, Indian frankincense

Useful Part: Resin

Habitation: Boswellia is native to Asia and Africa

This medicinal herb was used in the Indian Ayurvedic system of medicine for more than two thousand years. Prehistoric healers also used Boswellia to treat ailments such as diabetes, rheumatism, cardiovascular disorders, fever, and asthma. These days, it's often used to treat the pain of the joints and inflammation.

PRECAUTION: Boswellia may result in diarrhea and nausea if used in large dosages. People with severe kidney and liver disease should not use this herb and should be avoided by pregnant women

- **Herb**: Buchu

Scientific Name: Agathosma betulina

Family: Rutaceae

Common Names: Diosma, bookoo, Bucco, Buchu, boegoe

Useful Part: Leaves

Habitation: Buchu is indigenous to South Africa

This medicinal herb is commonly used as a diuretic and a stimulating tonic. It has also been used in the past to treat gout, kidney stones, and arthritis. Buchu is now often used to cure infections of the urinary tract. It's also being used externally for sprains and bruises.

- **Herb**: Burdock

Scientific Name: Arctium Lappa

Family: Asteraceae

Common Names: Burr, beggars buttons, Wild Burdock, Gobo

Useful Part: Seeds, leaves, and roots

Habitation: Burdock grows in China, Japan, Europe, and the United States

The ancient Greek used this medicinal herb for treating infections and wounds. Burdock possesses important minerals and vitamins and often used to cure digestive and liver problems, eczema, ulcers, psoriasis, and urinary tract infections. It is also used to boost stamina and energy. It possesses anti-bacterial and anti-fungal properties that make a perfect blood purifier and immune system booster.

PRECAUTION: Burdock is a great detoxifier and can intensify certain kinds of skin conditions before the start of the healing process. It might interfere with many prescription medicines, such as those for treating blood sugar ailments and diabetes. Nursing mother or pregnant women should consult their physician before using this herb.

- **Herb**: Butterbur

Scientific Name: Petasites hybridus

Family: Asteraceae

Common Names: Pestilence wort, coughwort, Common butterbur

Useful Part: Leaves, rhizomes

Habitation: Butterbur is native to Europe and Asia

This medicinal herb has been used traditionally to treat urinary problems, fever, coughs and to expel intestinal parasites. Today, butterbur is often used to treat migraine headaches and as an anti-inflammatory agent. It's often taken to reduce smooth muscle spasms. Several studies have established that butterbur is effective in lessening bronchial spasms in people with asthma and bronchitis.

- **Herb**: Calendula

Scientific Name: Calendula officinalis

Family: Asteraceae

Common Names: Cape Weed, poet's marigold, Pot marigold

Useful Part: Flowers

Habitation: Calendula is indigenous to the Mediterranean region.

Traditionally, this medicinal plant was used to treat open sores, cure jaundice, break fevers, induce menstruation and for liver and stomach problems. Calendula possesses anti-inflammatory and antiseptic properties and could be used externally to treat eczema and sunburn. Now it's commonly used externally to heal wounds and stimulate tissue repair.

PRECAUTION: Calendula is not safe to be consumed by pregnant women and nursing mother.

Do not take Calendula internally if pregnant or nursing.

- **Herb**: Cascara Sagrada

Scientific Name: Frangula purshiana

Family: Rhamnaceae

Common Names: sacred bark, Cascara buckthorn, California buckthory

Useful Part: Bark

Habitation: Cascara Sagrada is indigenous to the Pacific Northwest in North America

This medicinal plant was used by the Native Americans to treat constipation, hemorrhoids, jaundice, stomach upset, and colitis as well as a laxative. Cascara Sagrada is now often used as a laxative.

PRECAUTION: This herb is not found as safe to be consumed by the FDA. It's often too strong of a laxative and could result in severe stomach upset. A mild laxative like Psyllium is generally recommended. Not safe for pregnant women.

- **Herb**: Catnip

Scientific Name: Nepeta cataria

Family: Lamiaceae

Common Names: Catrup, catnep, Catmint, catswort,

Part Used: Leaves, Flowers

Habitation: Catnip is native to Europe and Asia

This medicinal herb was often used by medieval herbalists to treat bruises, scalp irritations, gas, restlessness, and coughs. Catnip is now commonly used to treat diarrhea, flu, fever, cold, colic, and upset stomach. It's sometimes being used as a mild laxative to treat allergies and inflammation.

PRECAUTION: Catnip should not be given to children, used by pregnant women and nursing mother as it might stimulate the uterus and lead to miscarriage. It is also not safe to smoke.

- **Herb**: Cat's Claw

Scientific Name: Uncaria tomentosa

Family: Rubiaceae

Common Names: Hawk's claw, Peruvian cat's claw

Useful Part: Root, bark,

Habitation: Cat's Claw is indigenous to Central and South America.

This medicinal herb has been used for centuries by the natives of Peru to treat ailments such as intestinal problems, ulcers, asthma, arthritis, bone pain, and urinary tract infections. Today, cat's claw is commonly used as an anti-inflammatory and immune system booster. It's also used to treat cancer and rheumatism.

PRECAUTION: Cat's claw should not be taken by nursing mother and pregnant women or be given to children.

- **Herb**: Cayenne

Scientific Name: Capsicum annuum

Family: Solanaceae

Common Names: Chili pepper, red pepper, capsicum

Useful Part: Fruit

Habitation: Cayenne is indigenous to tropical regions of America.

This medicinal plant was used by the Native American to cure infections and as a pain reliever. Cayenne was also used to aid digestion, treat arthritis, and toothache. It possesses anti-bacterial compounds that enhance blood flow and rich in antioxidants, minerals and vitamins' Cayenne is consumed by many people to maintain cardiovascular health.

PRECAUTION: Consuming large quantities of cayenne could result in stomach upset. Be careful when handling, as hot peppers like cayenne might irritate the skin.

- **Herb**: Chamomile

Scientific Name: Matricaria recutita

Family: Asteraceae

Common Names: Wild chamomile, German chamomile,

Useful Part: Oil and flower heads

Habitation: Chamomile is native to Europe, Africa, and Asia

Ancient Egyptians used this medicinal plant for chills and fever. Today, it's still in use globally. Chamomile is often used to treat flatulence, bloating heartburn, indigestion, colic, and to calm nervousness. It has antibacterial, antiseptic, antispasmodic, antifungal, and anti-inflammatory properties. Chamomile tea has been found as a reliever by some people suffering from peptic ulcers.

PRECAUTION: Chamomile might lead to allergic reactions in those sensitive to ragweed or other plants in the daisy family.

- **Herb**: Chaparral

Scientific Name: Larrea tridentata

Family: Zygophyllaceae

Common Names: Hediondilla, gobernadora, creosote bush, stinkweed

Useful Part: Twigs and leaves

Habitation: Chaparral is indigenous to Mexico and the U.S.

This medicinal herb was used by the Native Americans to treat diarrhea, bronchitis, flu, colds, intestinal and urinary tract problems. The twigs of chaparral were chewed to relieve toothaches. Nowadays, the plant is found to possess a ponent antioxidant and being studied as a potential remedy for cancer.

- **Herb**: Chaste Tree

Scientific Name: Vitex agnus-castus

Family: Verbenaceae

Common Names: Abraham's balm, agnus castus, chaste berry, monk's pepper, vitex

Useful Part: Fruits

Habitation: The chaste tree is indigenous to Western Asia and Southern Europe

This medicinal plant has been used for more than 2,500 years to treat gynecological troubles such as to relieve menstrual pain, promote normal menstruation and treat other menstrual conditions.

Today, chaste tree is still performing the same curative functions.

PRECAUTION: Do not take the chaste tree with any hormone medication and do not take during pregnancy.

- **Herb**: Chicory

Scientific Name: Cichorium intybus

Family: Asteraceae

Common Names: Coffeeweed, succory, wild succory

Useful Part: Whole herb

Habitation: Chicory is native to North America, Asia, and Europe.

The Native Americans commonly used this medicinal plant as a diuretic, nerve tonic, and blood purifiers. Nowadays, chicory is often used to treat indigestion and loss of appetite.

PRECAUTION: Chicory should not be consumed by people having gallstones.

- **Herb**: Cinnamon

Scientific Name: Cinnamonum verum

Family: Lauraceae

Common Names: Saigon cinnamon, Chinese cassia, ceylon cinnamon

Useful Part: Bark

Habitation: Cinnamon is indigenous to India, cultivated in Africa, South America and Indonesia.

This medicinal plant is commonly used to treat colds, indigestion, inflammation, and nausea. The essential oil of cinnamon has antibacterial, antifungal and antispasmodic properties.

- **Herb**: Clubmoss

Scientific Name: Lycopodium clavatum

Family: Lycopodiaceae

Common Names: Running pine, wolf's claw moss, ground pine, stag's horn moss

Useful Part: Whole plant

Habitation: Clubmoss is indigenous to the Southern and Northern Hemispheres

This medicinal herb has been used traditionally for more than 2,000 years. The druids used clubmoss for purgative and laxative The plant was used by the Native Americans to treat weakness of the body, fever, postpartum pain and to stop wound's bleeding. These days, clubmoss is commonly used to treat skin ailments, diarrhea, stomach upset, kidney and urinary disorders.

- **Herb**: Comfrey

Scientific Name: Symphytum officinale

Family: Boraginaceae

Common Names: Blackwort, knitbone, slippery root

Useful Part: Roots and leaves

Habitation: Comfrey is native to Asia and Europe

This medicinal plant was used by the ancient Greeks as a poultice to prevent bleeding. Comfrey was also consumed as a tea to treat bronchitis and diarrhea.

PRECAUTION: Comfrey should not be taken internally, though the ancient herbalists used it. Recent studies have revealed that it can cause liver damage.

- **Herb**: Cordyceps

Scientific Name: Cordyceps Sinensis

Family: Clavicipitaceae

Common Names: Cs-4, caterpillar fungus, Zhiling

Useful Part: Fruiting body

Habitation: Cordyceps mushrooms grow wild on the Himalayan Plateau

This medicinal plant has a long history of use in Chinese herbal tradition. Cordvceps is known to be an excellent tonic for endurance and building physical strength. It possesses a substance that dilates the lung's airway, supplying extra oxygen to the blood. That is why it's well-known with athletes. This herbal plant is also often used to treat bronchitis, cough, and asthma. It boosts the immune system and has anti-inflammatory properties.

- **Herb**: Dandelion

Scientific Name: Taraxacum officinale

Family: Asteraceae

Common Names: Priests Crown, wet weed, lion's tooth, fairy clock, blowball

Useful Part: Root, flowers, and leaves

Habitation: Dandelion is indigenous to Asia and Europe but grows all over the world

This medicinal plant was commonly used in ancient China as a detoxifying medication and potent diuretic. It was also often used to treat appendicitis, digestive disorders, breast inflammation and to stimulate the flow of milk. Dandelion was used by

Ancient Europeans to treat fever, diabetes, diarrhea, and eye problems.

- **Herb**: Dong Quai

Scientific Name: Angelica Sinensis

Family: Apiaceae

Common Names: Chinese angelica, danggui, tang-kuei

Useful Part: Root

Habitation: This herb is indigenous to China, Korea, and Japan

Dong Quai is commonly called female ginseng in China. Women use this medicinal herb as a therapy for menstrual cycle ailments and to treat menstrual pain and bleeding of the uterus. It's also used to relieve hot flashes, PMS, mood swings, and virginal dryness.

PRECAUTION: Dong Quai should not be taken during pregnancy as it can stimulate contractions of the uterus, hence leading to miscarriage.

- **Herb**: Echinacea

Scientific Name: Echinacea purpurea

Family: Asteraceae

Common Names: purple echinacea, coneflower, Purple coneflower

Useful Part: Flowers, leaves, and roots,

Habitation: Echinacea is indigenous to Eastern and Central North America.

This medicinal herb has been used to treat flu and colds. Echinacea is an excellent immune system booster. It has also been used to treat upper respiratory tract infection and sore throat. It's a great detoxifier and possesses antibiotic, anti-inflammatory, and antiviral properties.

- **Herb**: Fo-Ti

Scientific Name: Polygonum Multiflorum

Family: Polygonaceae

Common Names: Polygonum flower, climbing knotweed, Chinese cornbind, He Shou Wu, flowery knotweed,

Useful Part: Root

Habitation: Fo-Ti is indigenous to China

This medicinal herb has been used in China for thousands of years. Fo-Ti was often used to strengthen the lower back and knees. It could also be used to strengthen muscles, tendons, bones and to nourish blood. Fo Ti is very common with older men as it's found to be capable of turning their hair to their youthful color.

PRECAUTION: FoTi can cause diarrhea and stomach upset if large quantities are taken.

- **Herb**: Ginkgo Biloba

Scientific Name: Ginkgo biloba

Family: Ginkgoaceae

Common Names: Maidenhair tree, Yin-hsing, Ginkgo, bao gou

Useful Part: Seed and leaves

Habitation: Ginkgo biloba is indigenous to China but is also growing in Southern U.S, France, and Japan

This medicinal herb increases oxygen to the brain cells and enhances the flow of blood to the brain. Gingko Biloba is commonly used as a memory booster and effective cognitive enhancer. It has anti-coagulating materials which prevent blood clots formation. Consequently, it lessens the risk of stroke.

It also has flavonoids and terpenoids that protect the body from cell oxidation and free radical damage.

PRECAUTION: This herb could cause dizziness and headaches if taken in large quantities. Do not use Ginkgo when taking anti-depressants like SRRI or MAOI drugs.

- **Herb**: Gotu Kola

Scientific Name: Centella asictica

Family: Mackinlayaceae

Common Names: Luei gong gen, Brahmi, Centella, Indian pennywort

Useful Part: Stems and leaves,

Habitation: Gotu Kola grows in Asia, Australia, Africa, Madagascar, South, and North America

This medicinal herb has been used traditionally to ease congestion from upper respiratory infections, treat colds and heal wounds. Gotu kola is often used to treat loss of memory and varicose veins.

PRECAUTION: Gotu is not safe to be consumed by pregnant women, nursing mother and children without consulting your physician, as it may result in sensitivity to sunlight.

- **Herb**; Gynostemma

Scientific Name: Gynostemma Pentaphyllum

Family: Cucurbitaceae

Common Names: southern ginseng, Jiao Gu Lan, miracle herb, miracle tea, longevity herb

Useful Part: Leaves

Habitation: Gynostemma is indigenous to China, Korea, Japan, and Vietnam

This medicinal herb has been used to protect the body and mind against stress and to increase strength. Gynostemma is excellent for the digestive and cardiovascular system as well as boosting the immune system.

PRECAUTION: Do not take gyostemma with medicines or herbs that affect blood clotting and immune system suppression.

- **Herb**: Holy Basil

Scientific Name: Ocimum Sanctum

Family: Lamiaceae

Common Names: Kemangen, Surasa, Tulsi, Sacred basil, Tulasi

Useful Part: Stems and Leaves

Habitation: Holy Basil is indigenous to India

This medicinal herb is often used to reduce depression, anxiety, and stress. Holy basil promotes health and protects the mind and body positively. It's also found to improve memory and enhance cerebral circulation.

PRECAUTION; Holy basil is capable of thinning the blood, thus do not take with blood thinning medicines. Pregnant women and nursing mother should not use it without consulting a physician. Also, it should not be used by people having hypoglycemia.

- **Herb**: Kava

Scientific Name: Piper Methysticum

Family: Piperaceae

Common Names: Ava pepper, Kava, awa

Useful Part: Roots and rhizome

Habitation: Kava grows on the Pacific Islands

This medicinal herb has been used for thousands of years by the natives of the Pacific island as a natural treatment for anti-anxiety. Kava possesses a calming effect that sets people in good mood. Also, it has often been used to treat upset stomach, asthma, arthritis, urinary problems and as a diuretic. It's well-known in Germany where they often prescribed it as a treatment for anxiety disorders.

PRECAUTION: Kava is not safe to be used by pregnant women and nursing mother. Also, it may cause dizziness and dry mouth if taken excess dosages. Some studies suggested that kava may be harmful to the liver.

- **Herb**: Korean Ginseng

Scientific Name: Panax ginseng

Family: Araliaceae

Common Names: Asian ginseng, Asiatic ginger, the root of immortality, Oriental ginseng Manroot Korean ginseng

Useful Part: Root

Habitation: Korean ginseng is indigenous to China and Korea

This medicinal herb helps mind and body to deal with stress in a better way. Korean ginseng is an energizing herbal plant commonly used to improve mental ability, fight-off fatigue, increase strength and stamina. It also reduces cholesterol, helps to treat diabetes and depression as well as boosts immune system. Korean ginseng is best taken during winter due to its warming effect on the body.

PRECAUTION: Prolong use and higher dosages of Korean ginseng may be harmful to people with high blood pressure.

- **Herb**: Lemongrass

Scientific Name: Cymbopogon citratus

Family: Poaceae

Common Names: Citronella grass or gavati cha ha, tanglad, Silky heads, hierba Luisa, fever grass, barbed wire grass

Useful Part: Grass

Habitation: Lemongrass is indigenous to tropical India and Asia.

This medicinal herb is often used to treat conditions such as arthritis, fevers, body pain, gas, flu, nervous disorders, stomach problems, cancer and host of others. The tea of lemongrass helps to relax, reduce anxiety and enhances sound sleep. It could be used externally to treat skin troubles and keep the skin fresh and moist.

PRECAUTION: Do not use lemongrass during pregnancy as it contains uterine stimulating properties.

- **Herb**: Licorice Root, Chinese

Scientific Name: Glycyrrhiza Uralensis

Family: Legume

Common Names: Pink grass, beauty grass, Guo Lao, sweat herb, elf grass, sweet wood

Useful Part: Root

Habitation: Chinese licorice root is indigenous to Asia.

This herbal plant is well-liked in the Chinese traditional herbal system. Licorice root is added to numerous herbal formulas to enhance their effectiveness. It is a strong detoxifier.

PRECAUTION: Licorice root is not safe to be taken by people with high blood pressure or heart disease. It is also not safe to be used by nursing mother or during pregnancy.

- **Herb**: Lion's Mane

Scientific Name: Hericium erinaceus

Family: Hericiaceae

Common Names: Pom Pom, Monkey's Head, Bearded hedgehog, Hedgehog mushroom, Japanese yamabushitake, Bearded tooth, Old man's beard, Sheep's head, Bear's head, Hedgehog and Satyr's beard

Useful Part: Fruiting Body

Habitation: The Lion's mane mushroom thrives in Asia, Europe and parts of North America

This medicinal plant has been used as an immune system booster, to relieve depression and anxiety, promote digestive and colon health as well as improve memory. Lion's mane is also used to stimulate the synthesis of nerve growth factor and lower blood pressure. It's found to be an excellent curative for Alzheimer's and dementia disease.

- **Herb**: Lycium Fruit

Scientific Name: Lycium barbarum

Family: Solanaceae

Common Names: Wolfberry Goji

Useful Part: Fruit

Habitation: Lycium grows in Northwestern China and Tibet

This medicinal plant has been consumed In China for hundreds of years for its health-giving properties and good taste. Lycium berry is very nutritious as it provides minerals and vitamins to the body It also possesses antioxidant properties.

PRECAUTION: Do not consume Lycium when having low blood pressure.

- **Herb**: Maca

Scientific Name: Lepidium meyenii

Family: Brassicaceae

Common Names: Peruvian ginseng

Useful Part: Root

Habitation: Maca is indigenous to Peru

This herbal plant helps to manage stress. The root contains amino acids, plant sterols, good fats, minerals, and vitamins. The native of Peru discovered that taking maca root can improve physical strength and stamina, boost energy as well as libido. Athletes often use it. Nowadays, maca is commonly used for balancing the hormones and increasing energy.

PRECAUTION: Maca is not safe to be consumed during pregnancy. It has high iodine content so it's not safe to be taken by people with thyroid disease.

- **Herb**: Milk Thistle

Scientific Name: Silybum marianum

Family: Asteraceae

Common Names: Mary Thistle, Marian Thistle, Mediterranean Thistle, Silymarin

Useful Part: Seeds

Habitation: Milk Thistle is indigenous to Europe.

This medicinal herb has been used to protect the gallbladder and liver. Milk thistle is also often used to treat cancer and detoxify the blood.

- **Herb**: Maitake

Scientific Name: Grifola frondosa

Family: Meripilaceae

Common Names: Shelf Fungi, Hen of the Woods, King of Mushrooms, Dancing Mushroom, Cloud Mushroom, Grifola

Useful Part: Root

Habitation: Maitake is indigenous to Japan and China

This herbal plant contains high quantities of antioxidants, minerals, and vitamins. Maitake is often used to treat autoimmune disorders and cancer

- **Herb**: Rhodiola

Scientific Name: Rhodiola Rosea

Family: Crassulaceae

Common Names: Aaron's rod, Roseroot, Arctic Rose, Golden Root, Arctic Root,

Useful Part: Root

Habitation: Rhodiola is indigenous to Siberia

This herbal plant is well-liked by the Russian athletes and astronauts because of its ability to improve physical strength and endurance. Rhodiola is often used to improve memory and mental alertness. It's also a great anti-depressant and protects the body from all sorts of stress.

- **Herb**: Saw Palmetto

Scientific Name: Serenoa repens

Family: Palmae

Common Names: American dwarf palm tree, cabbage palm, sabal Fructus, Sabal palm, palmetto berry

Useful Part: Fruit

Habitation: Saw Palmetto grows in the islands of the Southeastern United States and West Indies

This herbal plant is popularly used by men above 40 years. Saw palmetto is commonly taken to treat Benign Prostatic Hyperplasia (BPH) and its symptoms, such as the frequent and painful urination. It has also been used to treat male pattern baldness by decreasing levels of the dihydrotestosterone (DHT) in the body. Baldness is believed to be caused by excessive DHT in the body.

PRECAUTION: Saw palmetto should not be taken with blood thinning medicines. Also, it should not be used if having ulcer, hemophilia or planning to have surgery as it may add to the risk of bleeding

- **Herb**: Schizandra

Scientific Name: Schizandra Chinensis

Family: Schisandraceae

Common Names: Magnolia vine Schisandra, Wu Wei Zi, Omicha, Five flavor berry

Useful Part: Fruit

Habitation: Schizandra is indigenous to northern China

This medicinal herb is often consumed to manage physical and mental stress. Schizandra is full of nutrition and gives extra energy.

PRECAUTION: Do not take Schizandra if you have a high brain (intracranial) pressure, peptic ulcer, epilepsy or gastroesophageal reflex disease (GERD).

- **Herb**: Shilajit

Scientific Name: Asphaltum

Common Names: Vegetable Asphalt, Mineral Pitch

Useful Part: The resin

Habitation: Shilajit can be native to Nepal, Tibet, and the Himalayan area.

This herbal plant contains minerals and vitamins good for overall health. Shilajit contains many vitamins and minerals and is often taken to increase longevity.

PRECAUTION: Shilajit is not safe to be used by pregnant women, nursing mother, and children. Do not use it if you have gout illness as it may increase uric acid in the body.

- **Herb**: Siberian Ginseng

Scientific Name: Eleutherococcus senticosus

Family: Araliaceae

Common Names: Eleuthero, Siberian ginseng

Useful Part: Root

Habitation: Siberian Ginseng is indigenous to Korea, China, and Russia

This medicinal herb has been found to be a great energizer and stress relief. Siberian ginseng has been used for centuries as an invigorating tonic herb. It's capable of normalizing and balancing the body. It was well-liked by the Russian athletes and cosmonauts for its ability to protect the mind and body from stress and improve the capability for hard physical and mental work.

PRECAUTION: Siberian Ginseng is not safe to be consumed by people with high blood pressure.

- **Herb**: Skullcap

Scientific Name: Scutellaria lateriflora

Family: Lamiaceae

Common Names: Blue pimpernel, helmet flower, hoodwort, mad dog, Quaker bonnet

Useful Part: The whole plant

Habitation: Skullcap grows in Asia, Canada, Europe, and the United States

This medicinal herb is capable of reducing nervousness and anxiety. It's commonly referred to as nature's tranquilizer. Skullcap has been used to aid sleep, treat low blood pressure and cholesterol, and relieve muscle pain and twitches. The plant also has anti-inflammatory properties and it's being used to treat joint pain and arthritis.

PRECAUTION: Skullcap should not be taken during pregnancy as it may cause miscarriage. Taken high quantity may result in liver damage.

- **Herb**: St. John's Wort

Scientific Name: Hypericum perforatum

Family: Hypericaceae

Common Names: Klamath weed, amber, hard hay Johnswort, goat weed

Useful Part:

Habitation: St. John's Wort grows in Australia, Europe, and The United States

This herbal plant is a great anti-depressant. It's commonly used to treat anxiety and depression. St. John's Wort works as a Selective Serotonin Reuptake Inhibitor (SSRI), as it permits the flow of serotonin. Thus makes you feel less anxious and depressed. This herb contains antiviral properties and could be used externally to treat wounds.

PRECAUTION: St. John Wort can aggravate sunburn in people with fair skin

- **Herb**: Suma

Scientific Name: Pfaffia paniculata

Family: Amaranthaceae

Common Names: Brazilian ginseng, Para Todo

Useful Part: Root

Habitation: Suma root is native to Ecuador, Brazil, Latin America, Panama, Peru, and Venezuela

This herbal plant is commonly called ginseng because of its ability to increase stamina and strength. It is great for lessening the ailing effects of stress. Suma is often taken for balancing the hormones and strengthen the adrenal glands. It has minerals, vitamins, and anti-inflammatory properties. It also possesses germanium that could boost the immune system.

PRECAUTION; Taken large dosages of Suma may cause nausea.

- **Herb**: Turmeric

Scientific Name: Curcuma longa

Family: Zingiberaceae

Common Names: Haridra, Jiang Huang, Indian saffron

Useful Part: Root

Habitation: Turmeric is indigenous to India

This herbal plant is known for its strong antioxidant called curcumin which makes it a good liver detoxifier.

PRECAUTION: Taking a large amount of turmeric can cause nausea, heartburn, and stomach upset. Nursing mother and pregnant women should not take it.□

Herb: Valerian

Scientific Name: Valerian officinalis

Family: Valerianaceae

Common Names: Amantilla, Set Well, English Valerian, Fragrant Valerian, Vandal Root St. George's Herb

Useful Part: Root

Habitation: Valerian is indigenous to Asia, North America, and Western Europe

This herbal plant has been used to relieve stress and as a remedy for insomnia as well as to treat anxiety. Valerian active ingredients increase the production for gamma aminobutyric acid (GABA) which is excellent for refreshing the brain.

PRECAUTION: Do not take valerian during pregnancy and don't give to children

CONCLUSION

As herbal plants are natural products they are almost free from side effects, they are locally available, eco-friendly and comparatively safe. Traditionally there are numerous herbal plants used for the diseases associated with different seasons. There is the necessity to promote them to save the human lives.

These medicinal herbs are nowadays the symbol of wellbeing in contrast to the synthetic medicines that are considered as dangerous to human's health and surroundings. Though herbal products had been valued for their aromatic, flavoring and medicinal qualities for hundreds of years, the synthetic products of present age exceeded their significance, for a while. Nevertheless, the blind reliance on synthetic has ended and people are now going back to the naturals with the hope of security and safety. It is time to promote them across the globe.